This **SeeMeDo**™ book belongs to:

_____

I Can Move!

Written by
Monica Lounsbery, PhD
&
Thom McKenzie, PhD

Art by
Tom Racine

Dedication

This book is dedicated to Tori and Payne Lounsbery; to Katie and Carly Racine--the greatest art the Artist will ever create; and to all children and their families.

Together, may we succeed in making physical activity an easy choice in homes, schools, and communities.

About the Authors

Drs. Monica Lounsbery and Thom McKenzie are internationally recognized educators and researchers who have spent decades studying physical activity.

With people becoming increasingly sedentary, Monica and Thom are focusing on Moving People More by developing a multi-division, multi-media effort to help people engineer physical activity back into their daily lives.

"I Can Move" is an Active Book

We wrote "I Can Move" to promote children and adults reading while moving together. Find a safe, open space and have a great time reading and moving!

For Parents, Guardians and Teachers

Physical activity contributes to children's overall health, including cardiovascular, muscle, bone, and intellectual development as well as reduced risk of obesity. Unfortunately, most children and adults are not active enough. Research shows that when children are at home they spend most of their time indoors, and being indoors is associated with long periods of sitting. Research also shows that activity levels of parents and children are related, and that adults often unknowingly suppress children's physical activity.

The 2008 *Physical Activity Guidelines for Americans* recommend that children should engage in at least 60 minutes of physical activity every day. They should avoid long bouts of sitting and move vigorously and play actively several times throughout the day.

"I Can Move" shows children being physically active indoors and outdoors at home and adults and children being active together. We hope that you enjoy the book and implement the research-based messages in it. We wish you the best in finding creative ways to make homes and schools active.

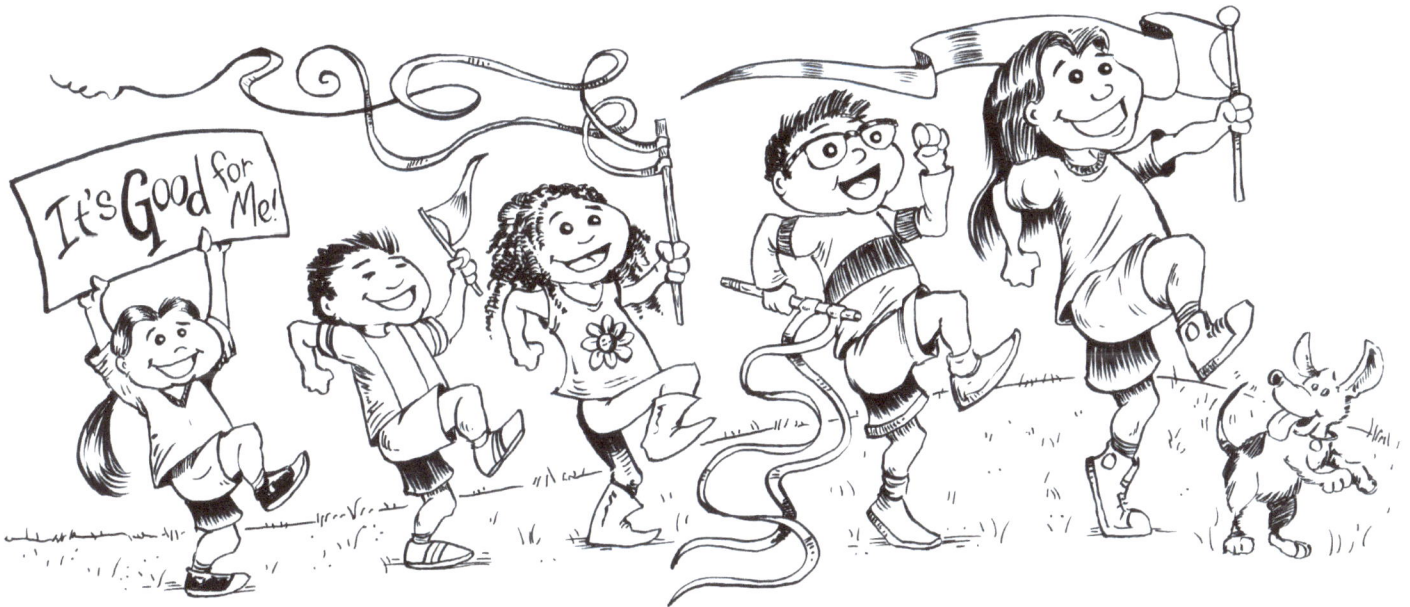

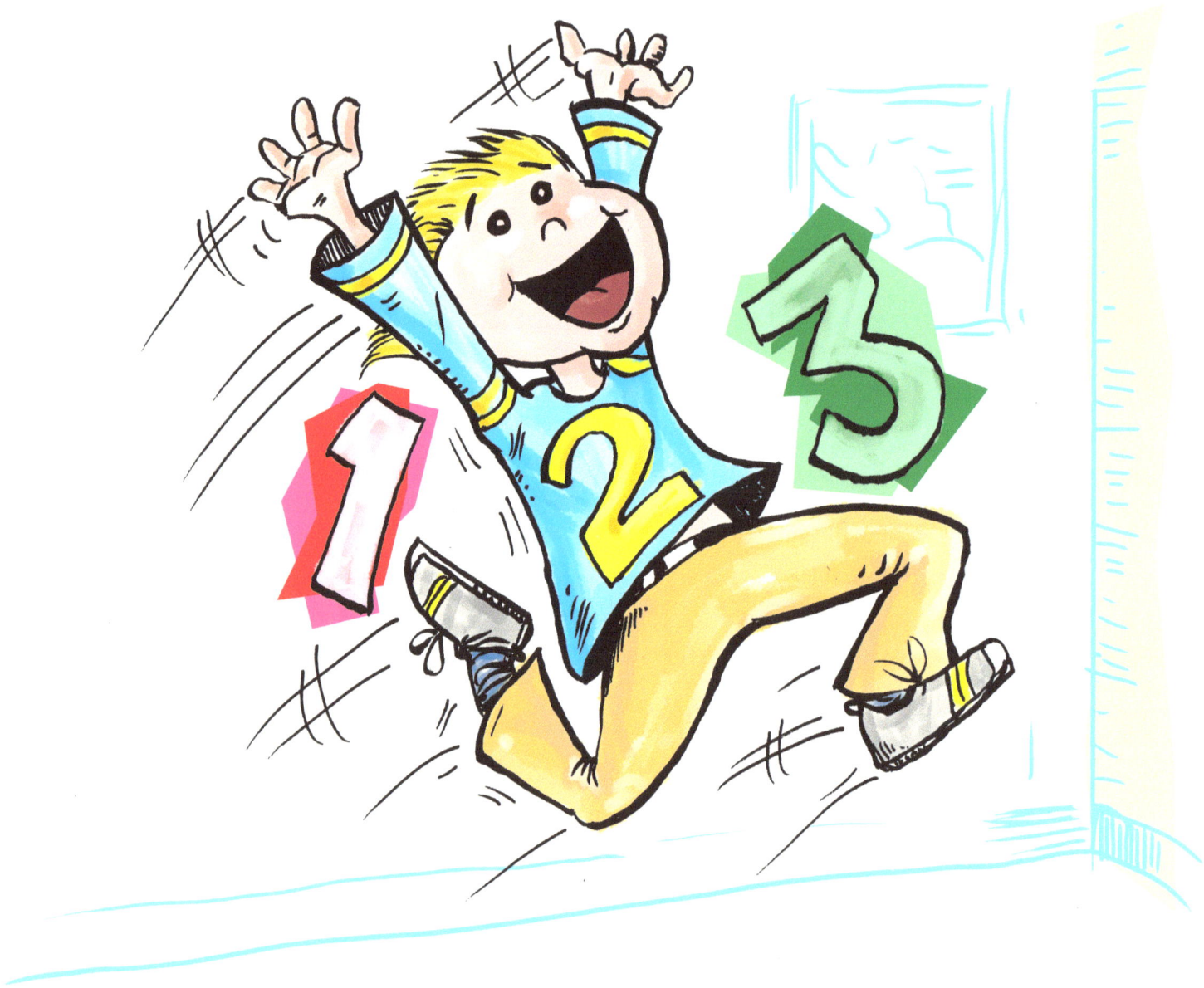

I can move!
Jump! One, Two, Three!

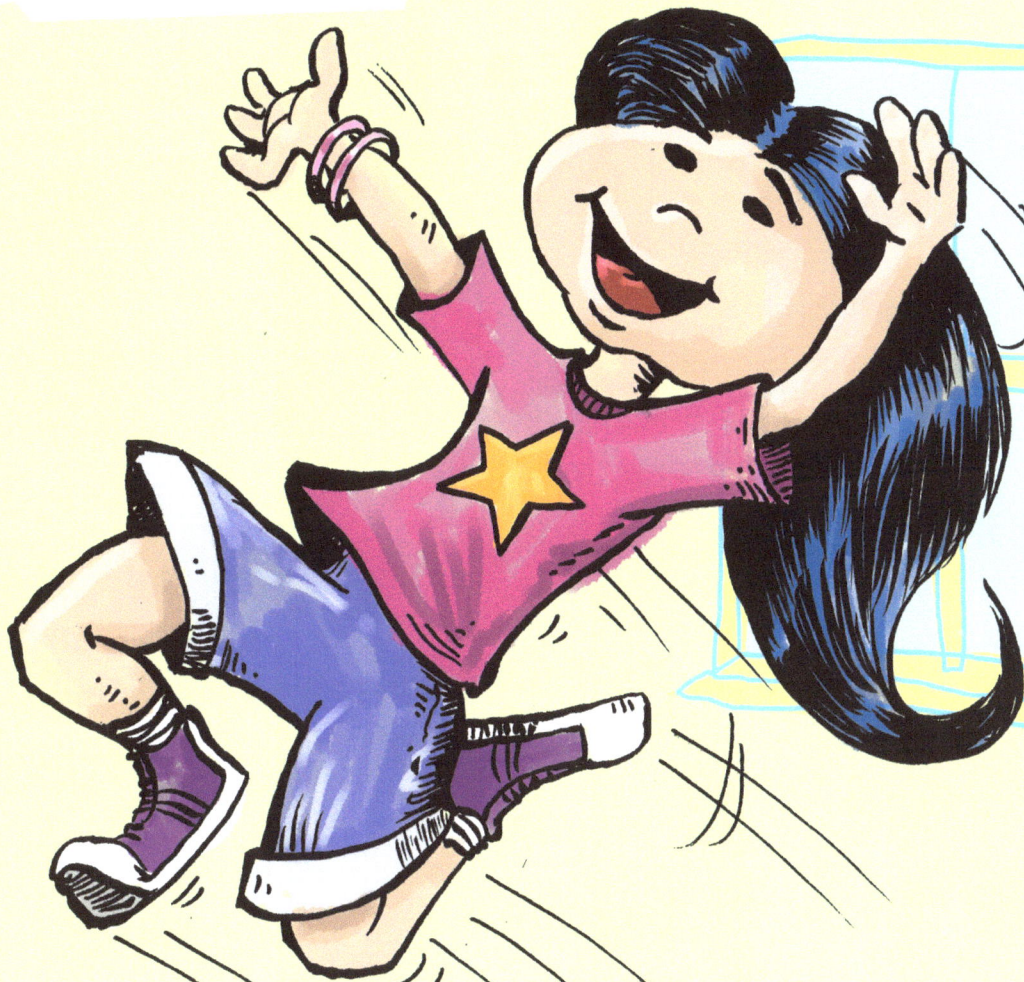

Shout out loud,
"It's good for me!"

2

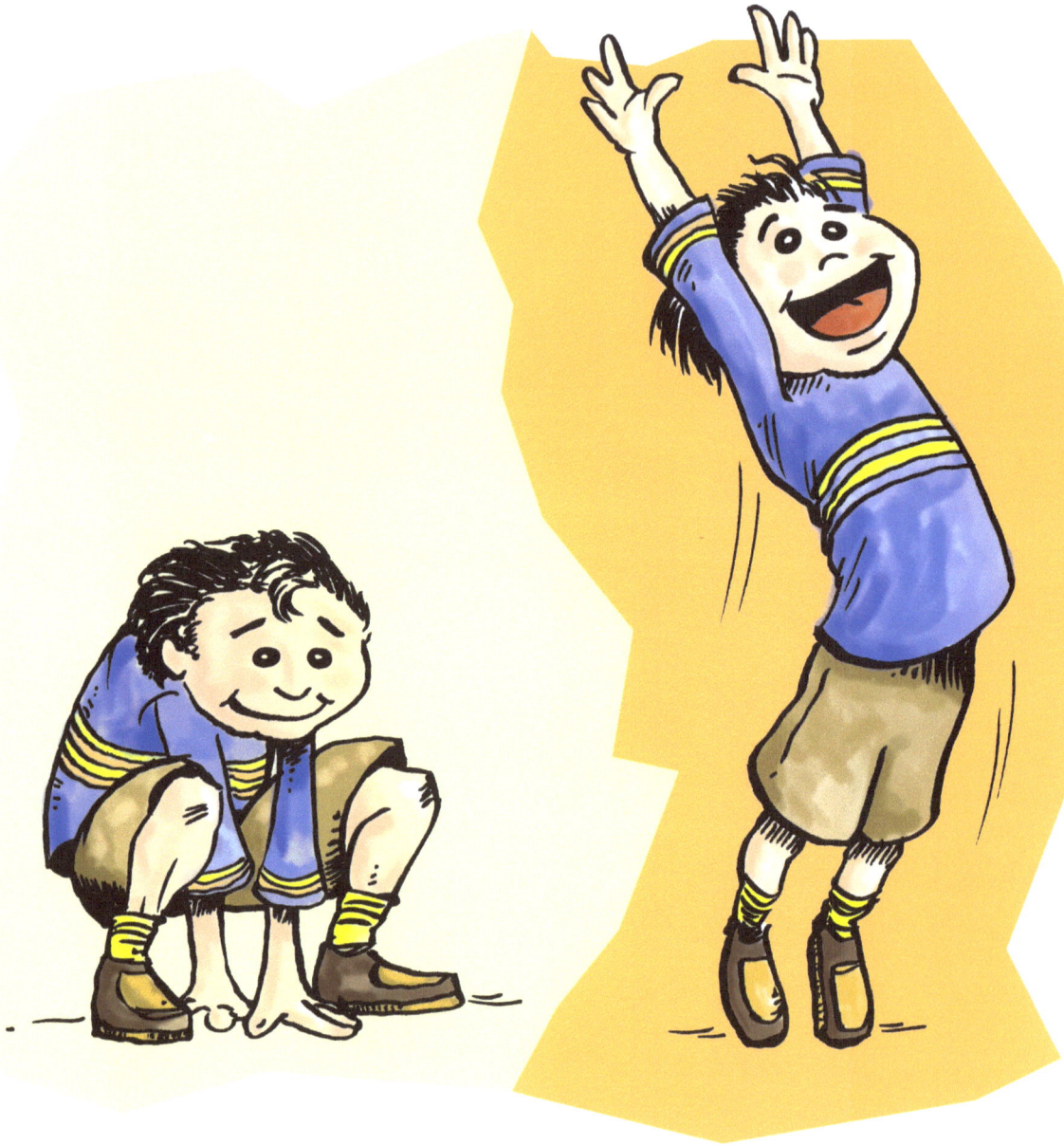

I crouch to the ground,
Then stretch up high.

3

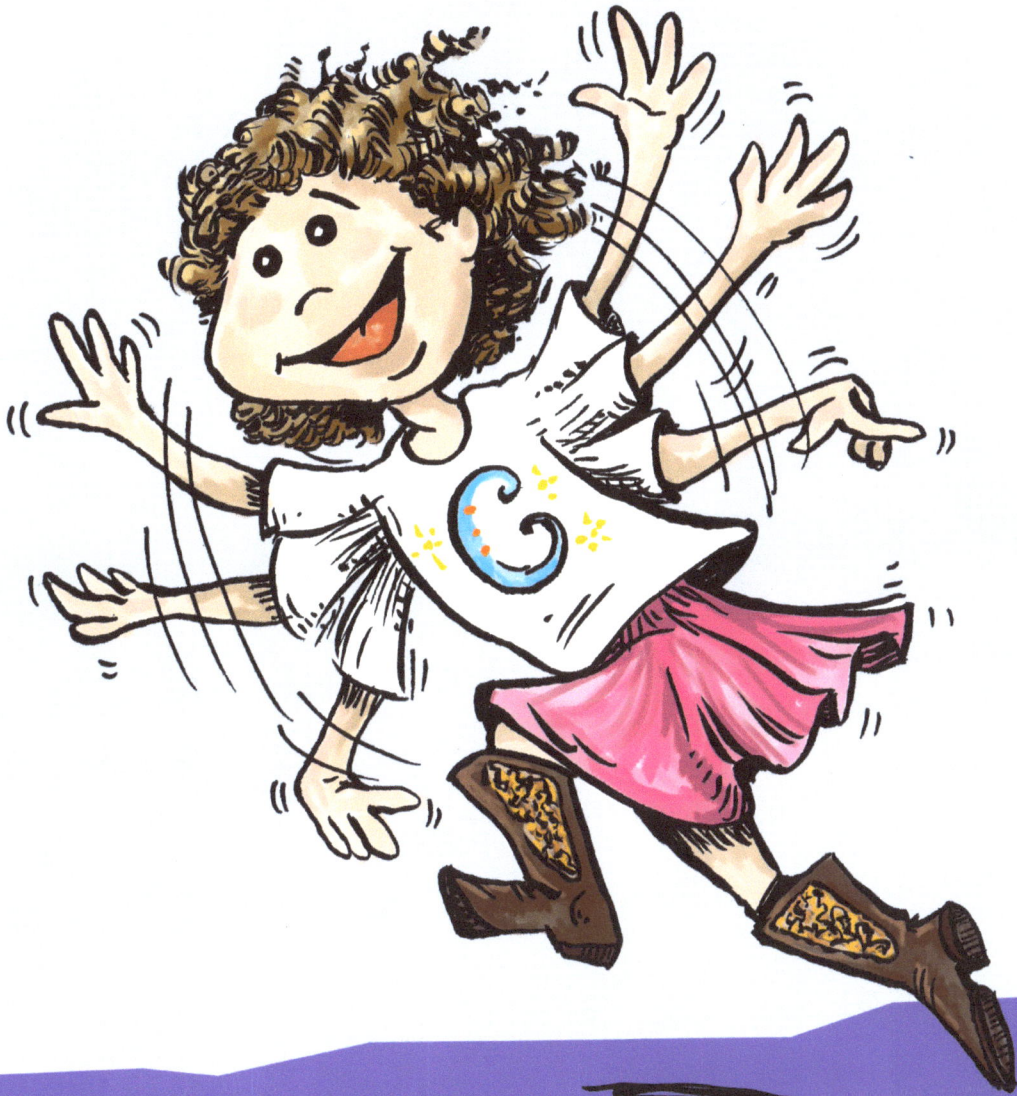

I flap my arms,
Watch me fly!

4

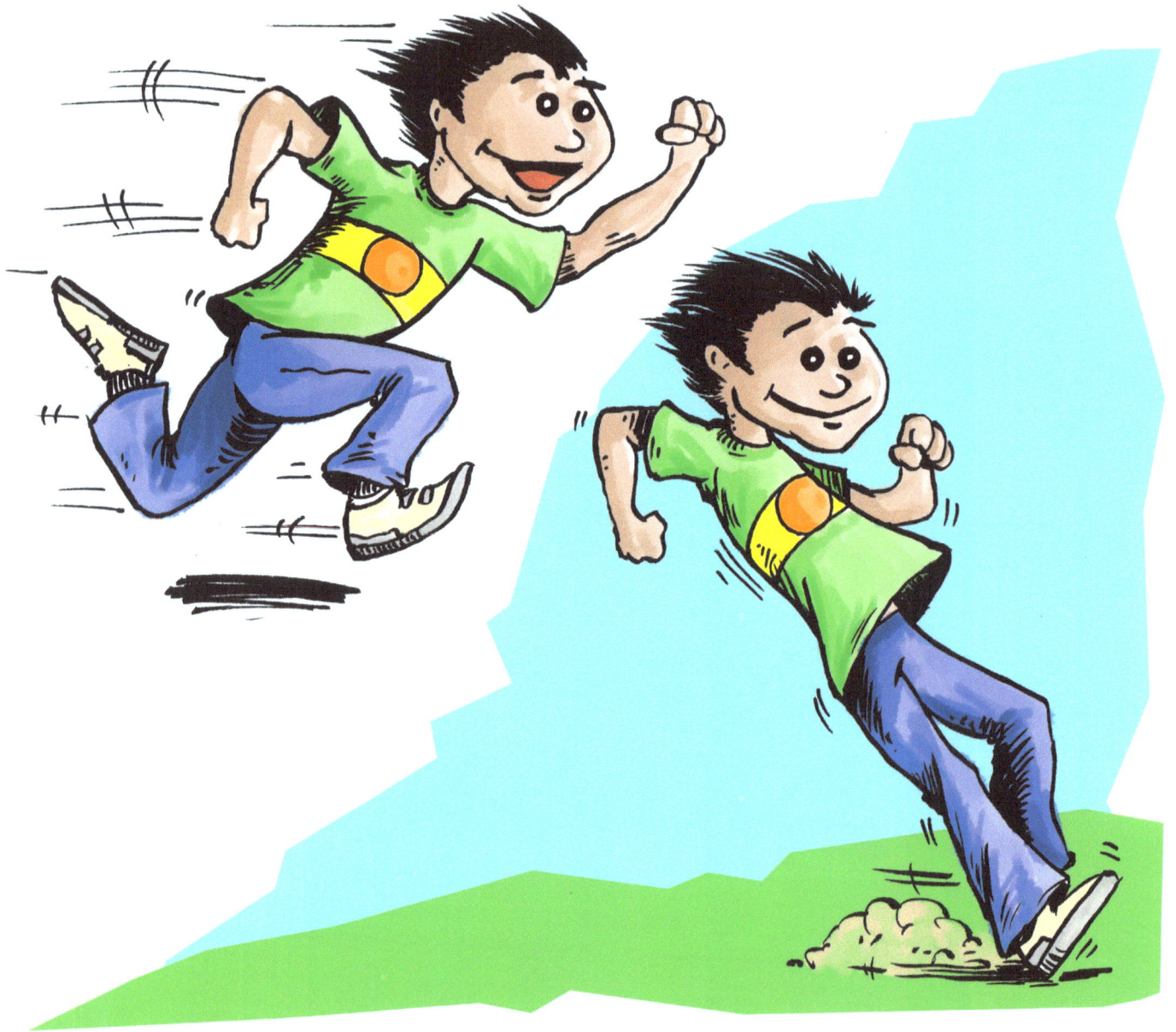

I run, run, run--
Then stop and go.

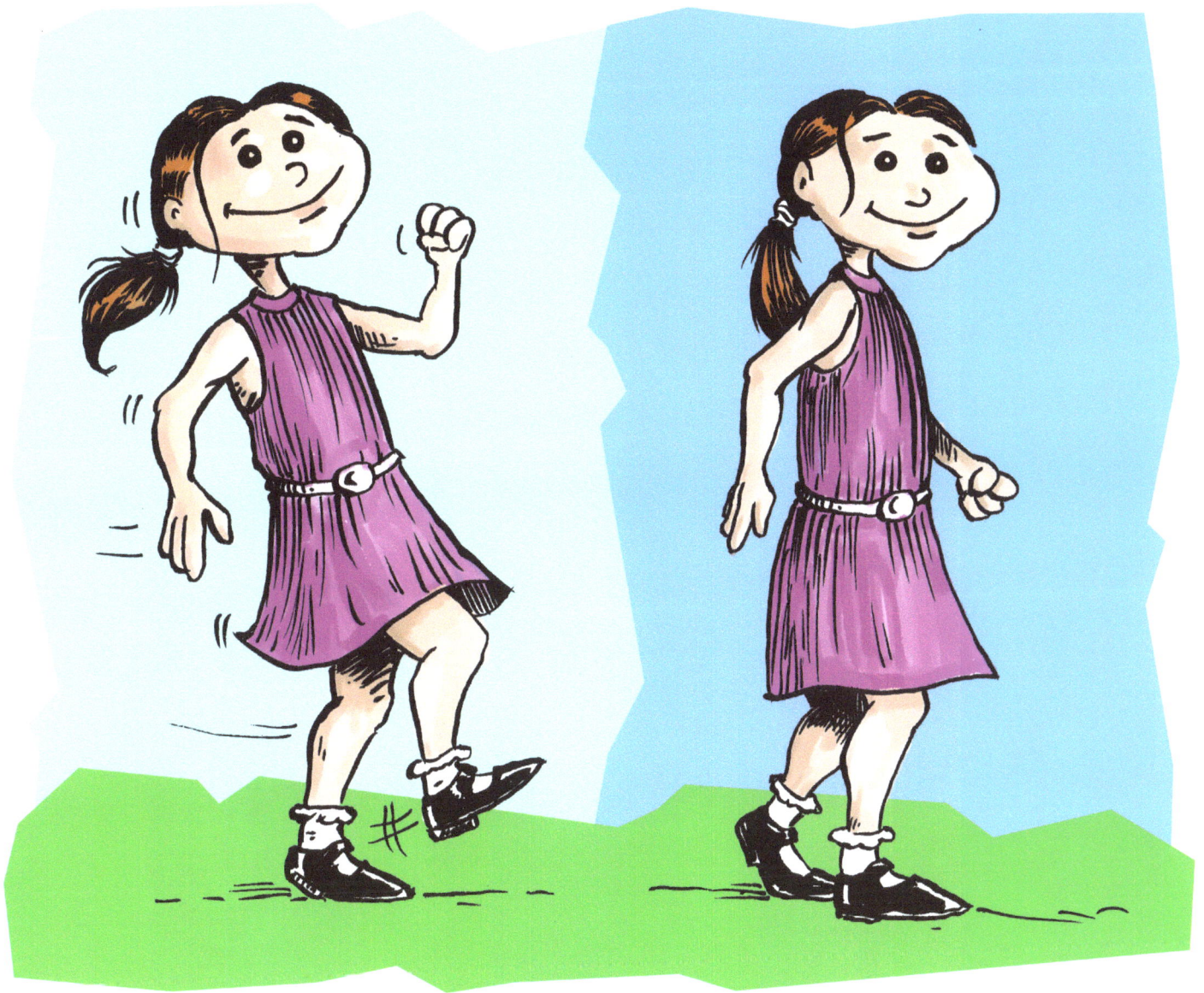

I walk real fast, and then real slow.
I can move, watch my show!

6

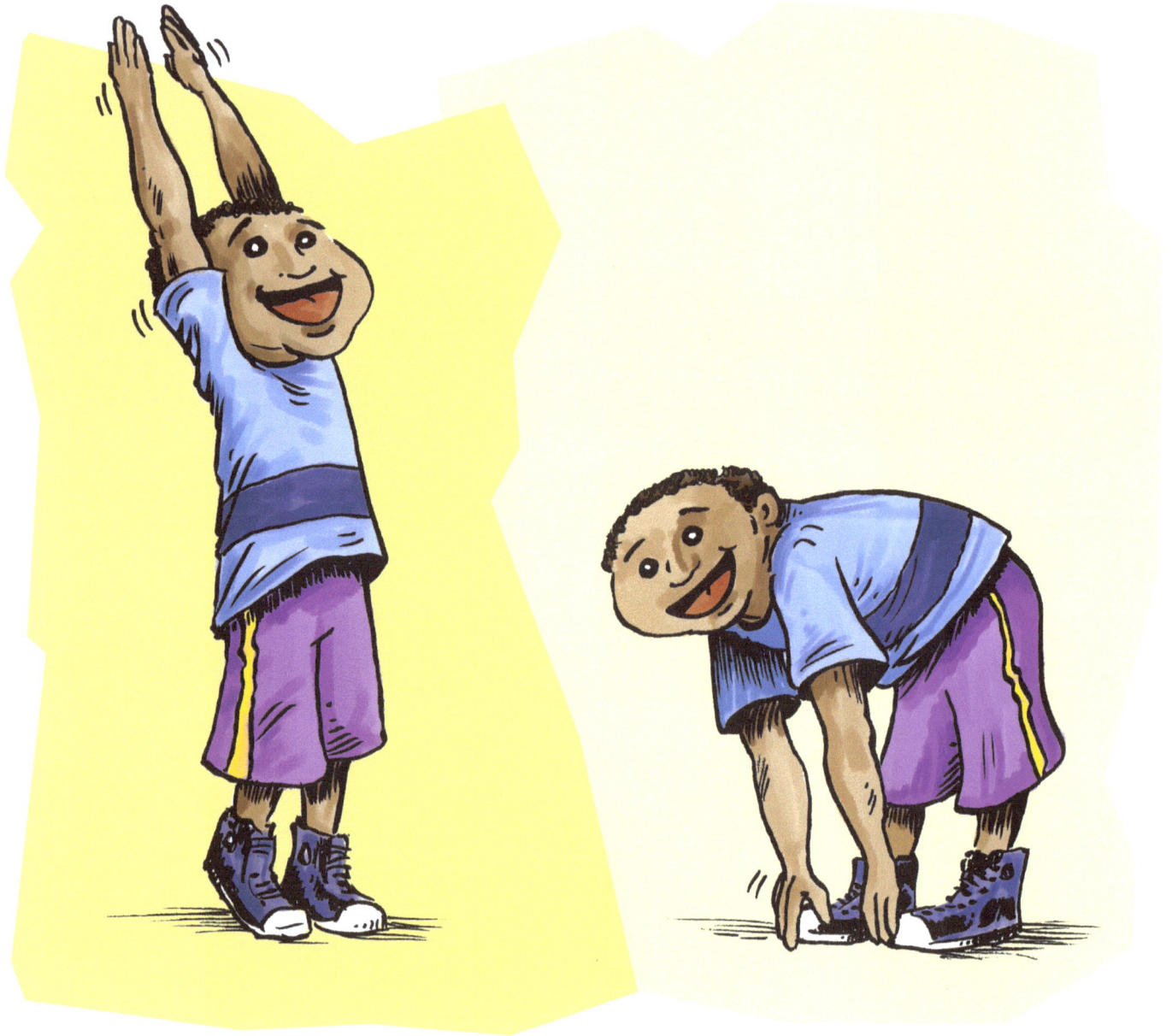

Moving is good. Moving is fun.
Moving is a ***must*** for everyone!

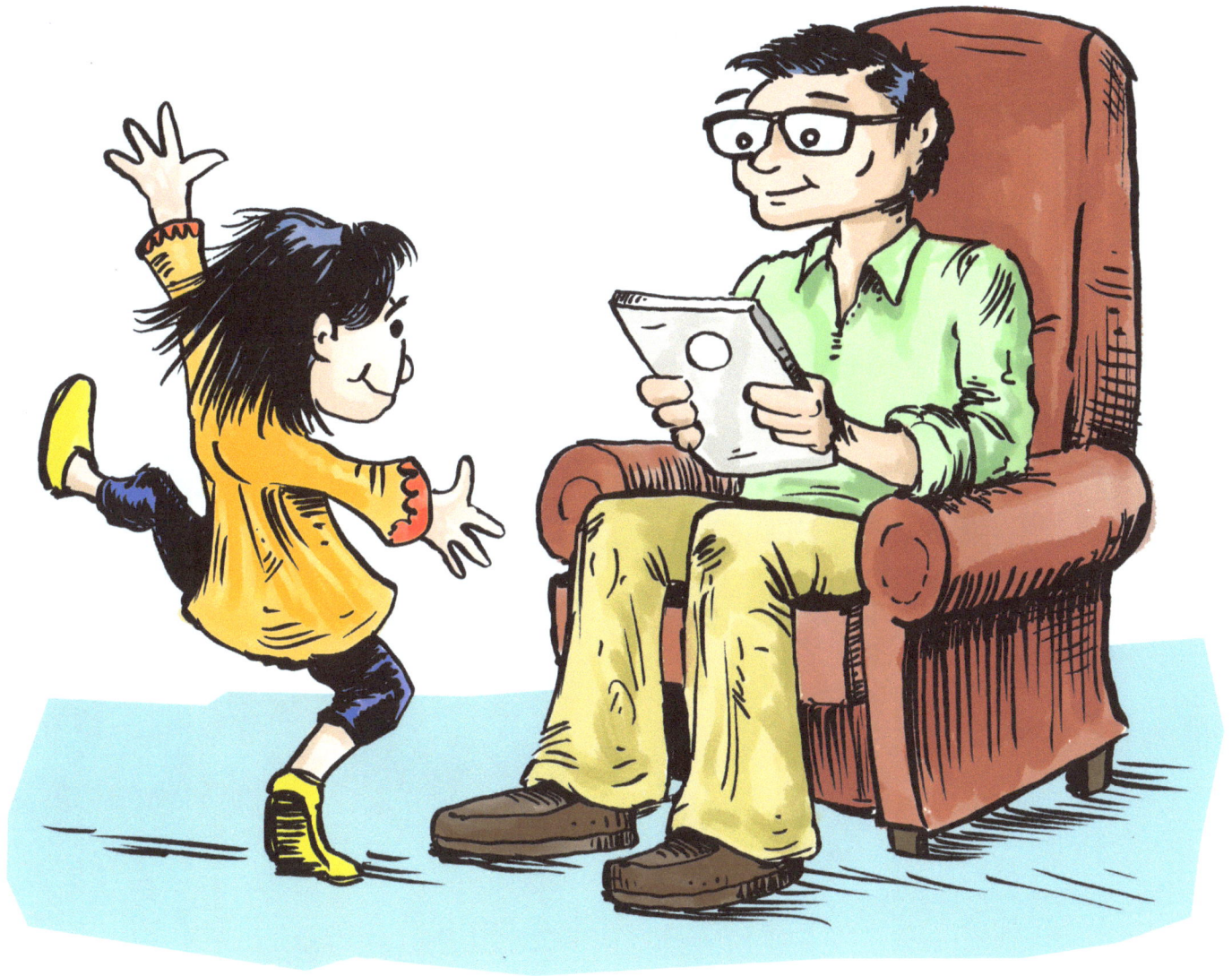

I need to move at least an hour a day.
I can move while I learn and I play!

8

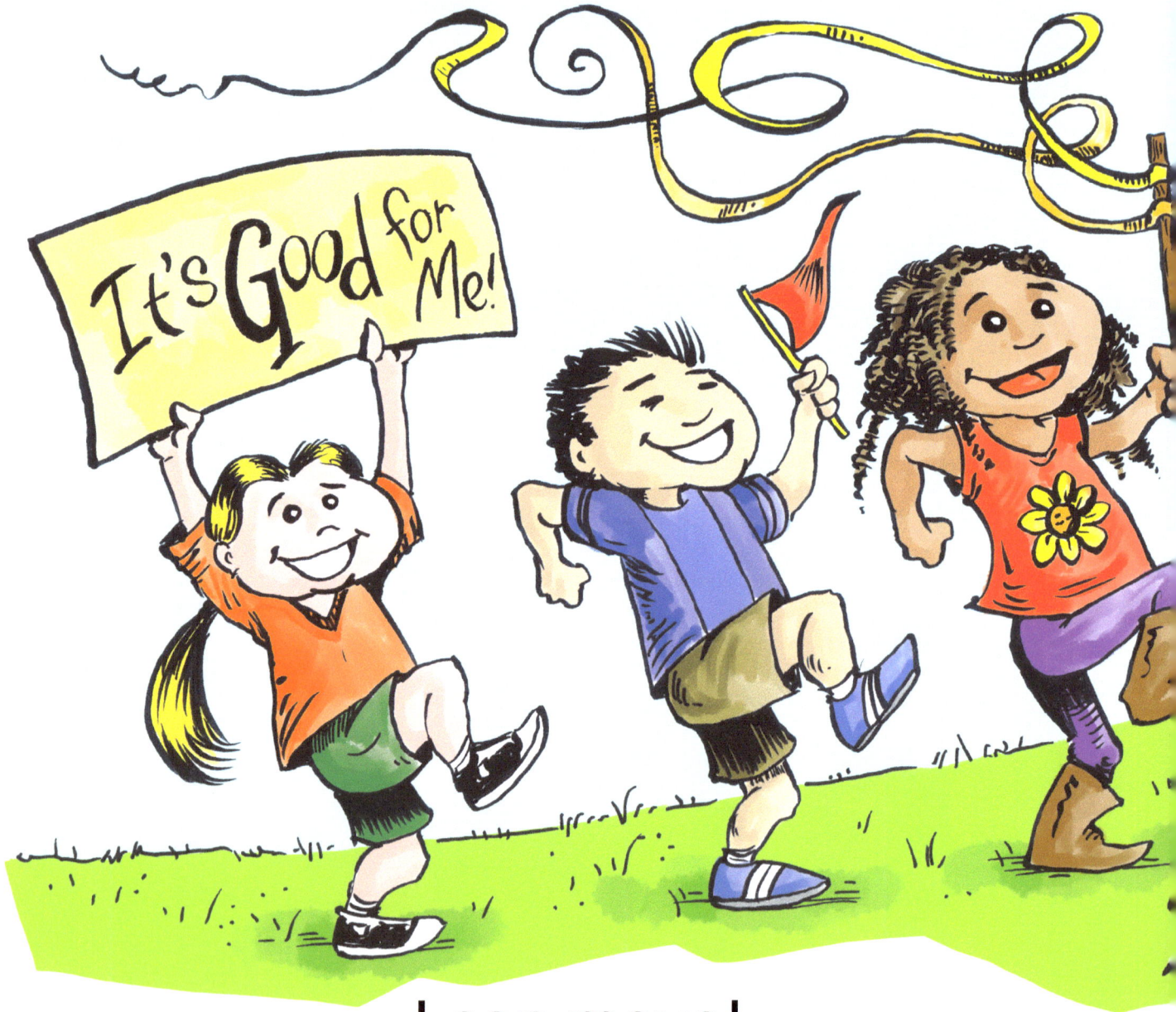

It's Good for Me!

I can move!
March! One, Two, Three!

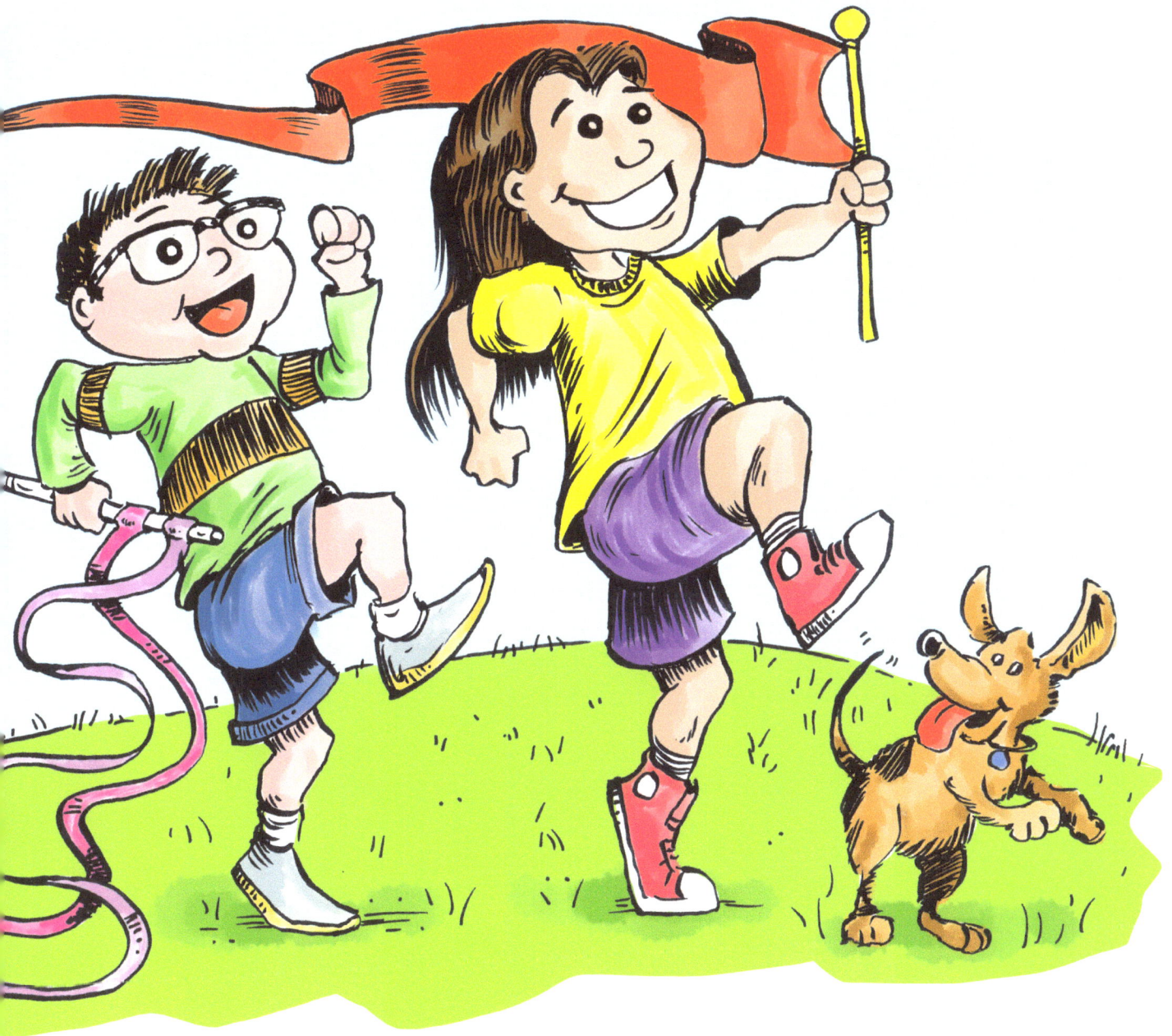

Shout out loud,
"It's good for me!"

10

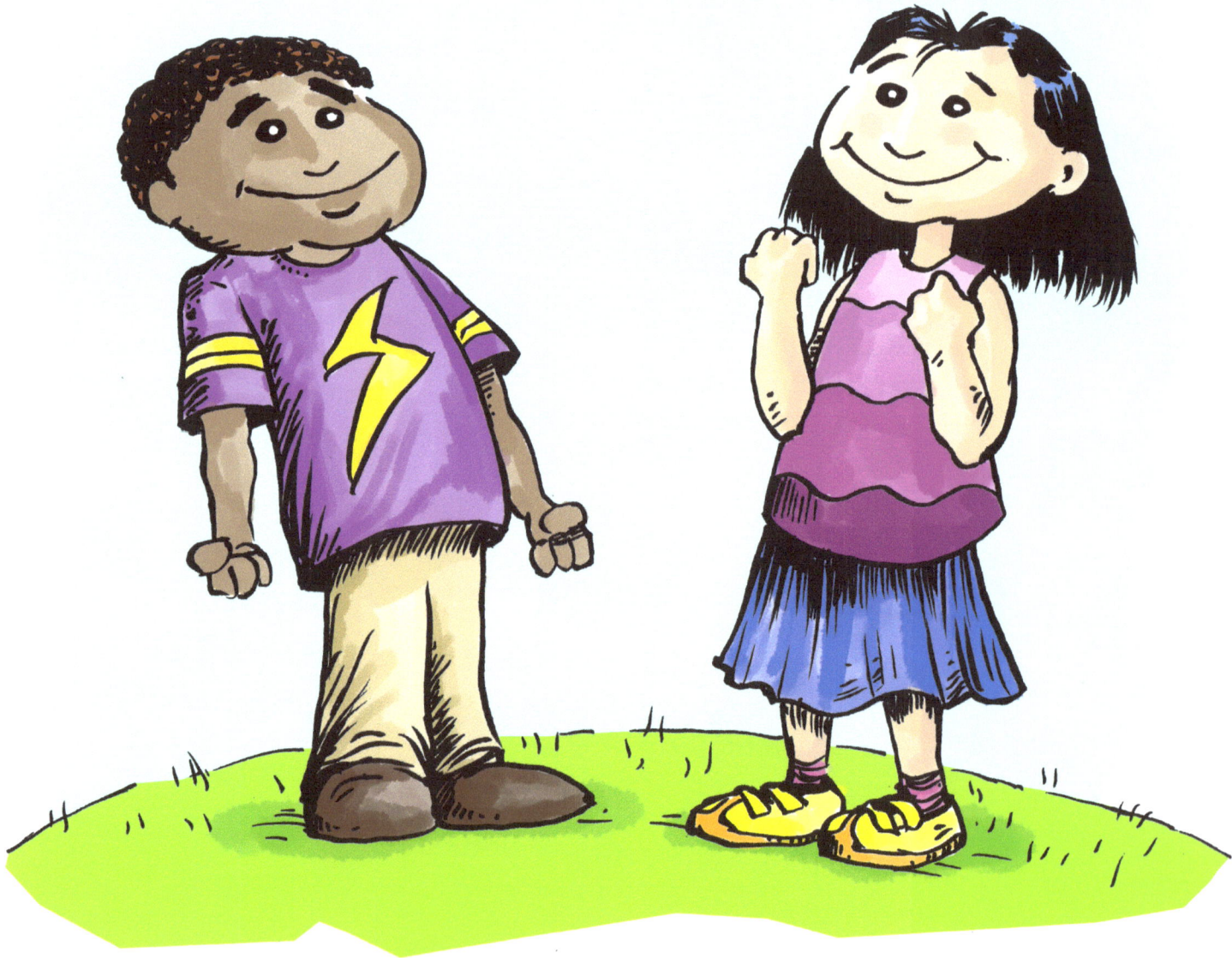

I curl both arms--
Up and down.

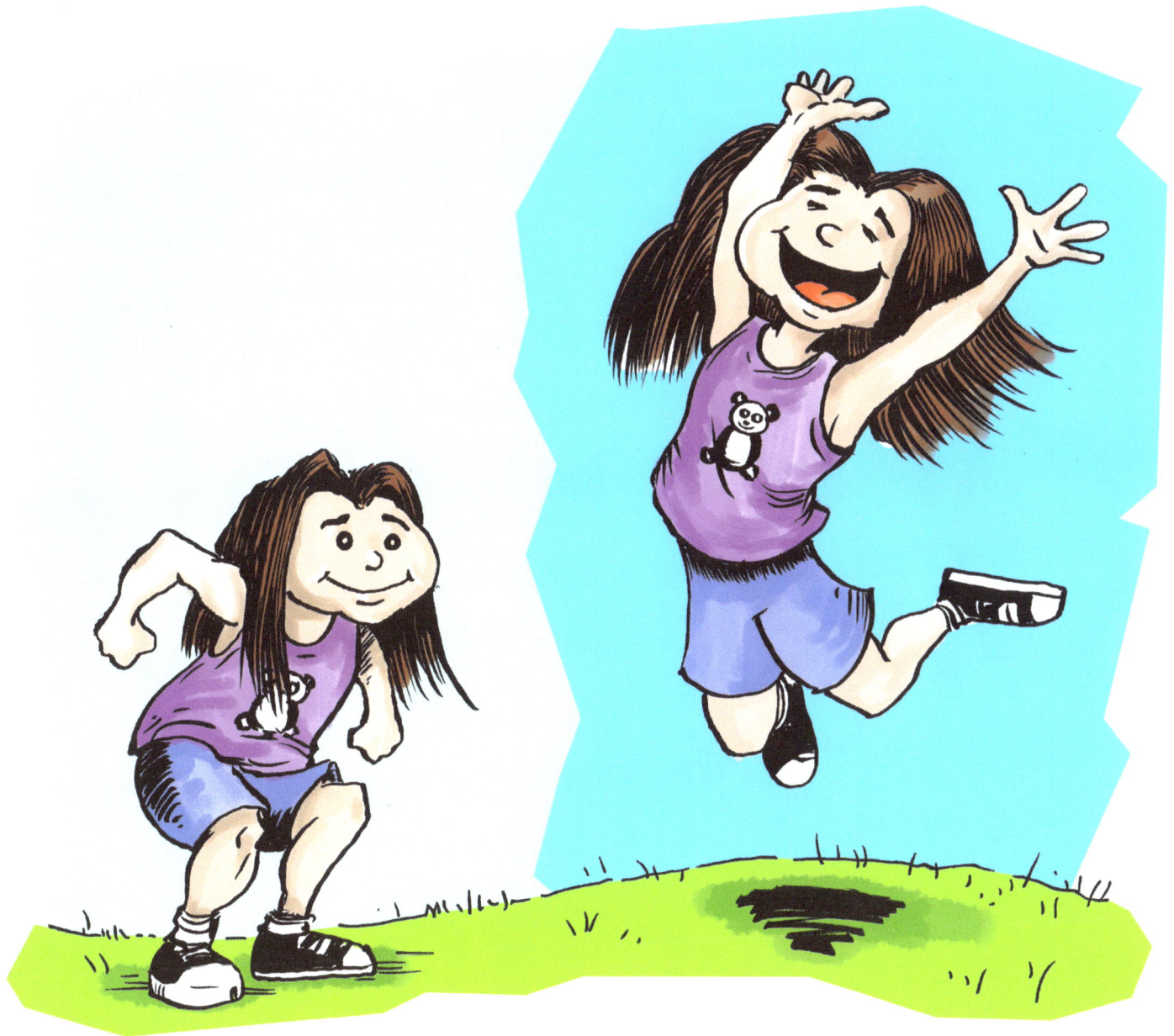

Bend my knees,
Jump off the ground!

12

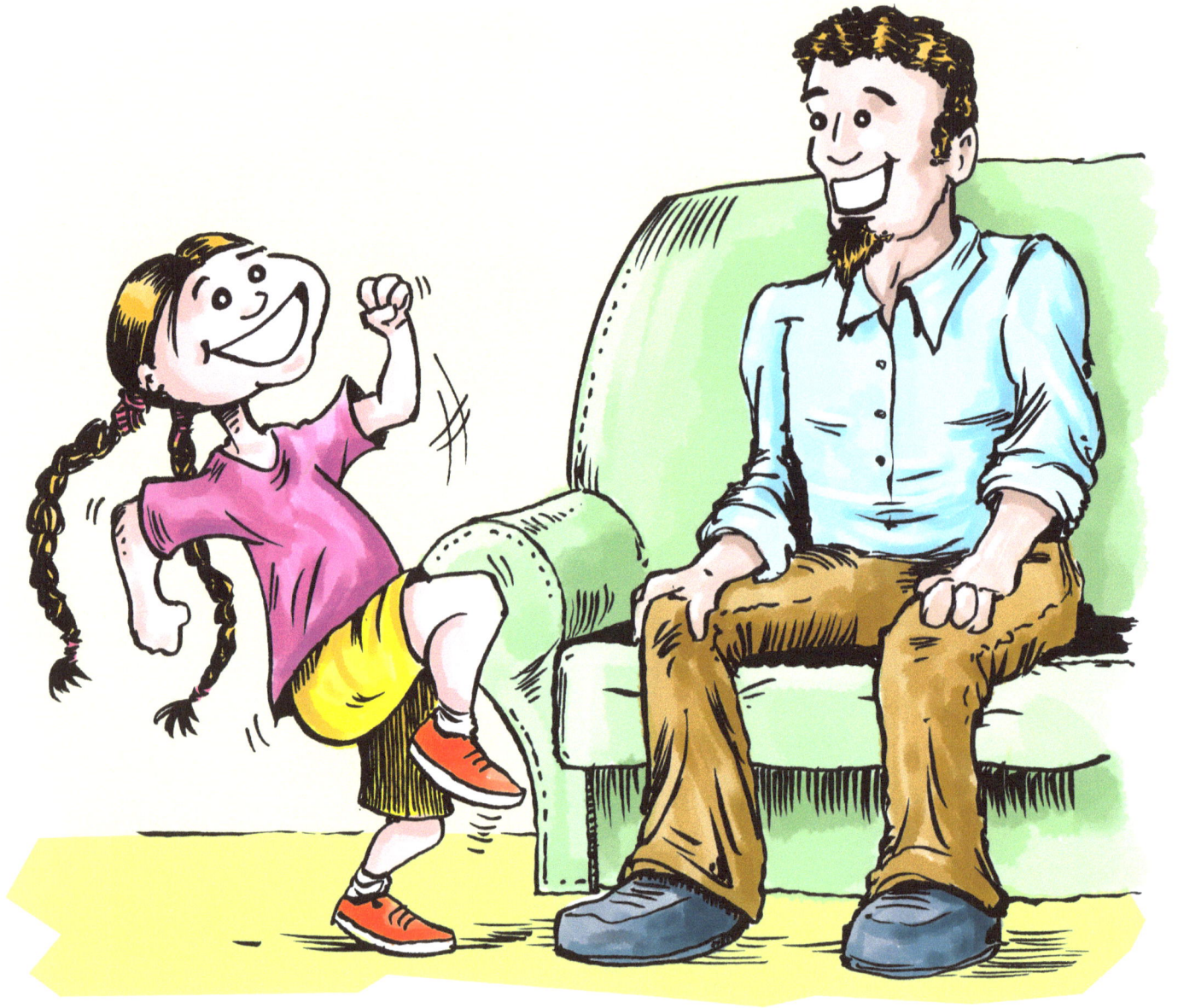

I step forward,
Then lift one knee.

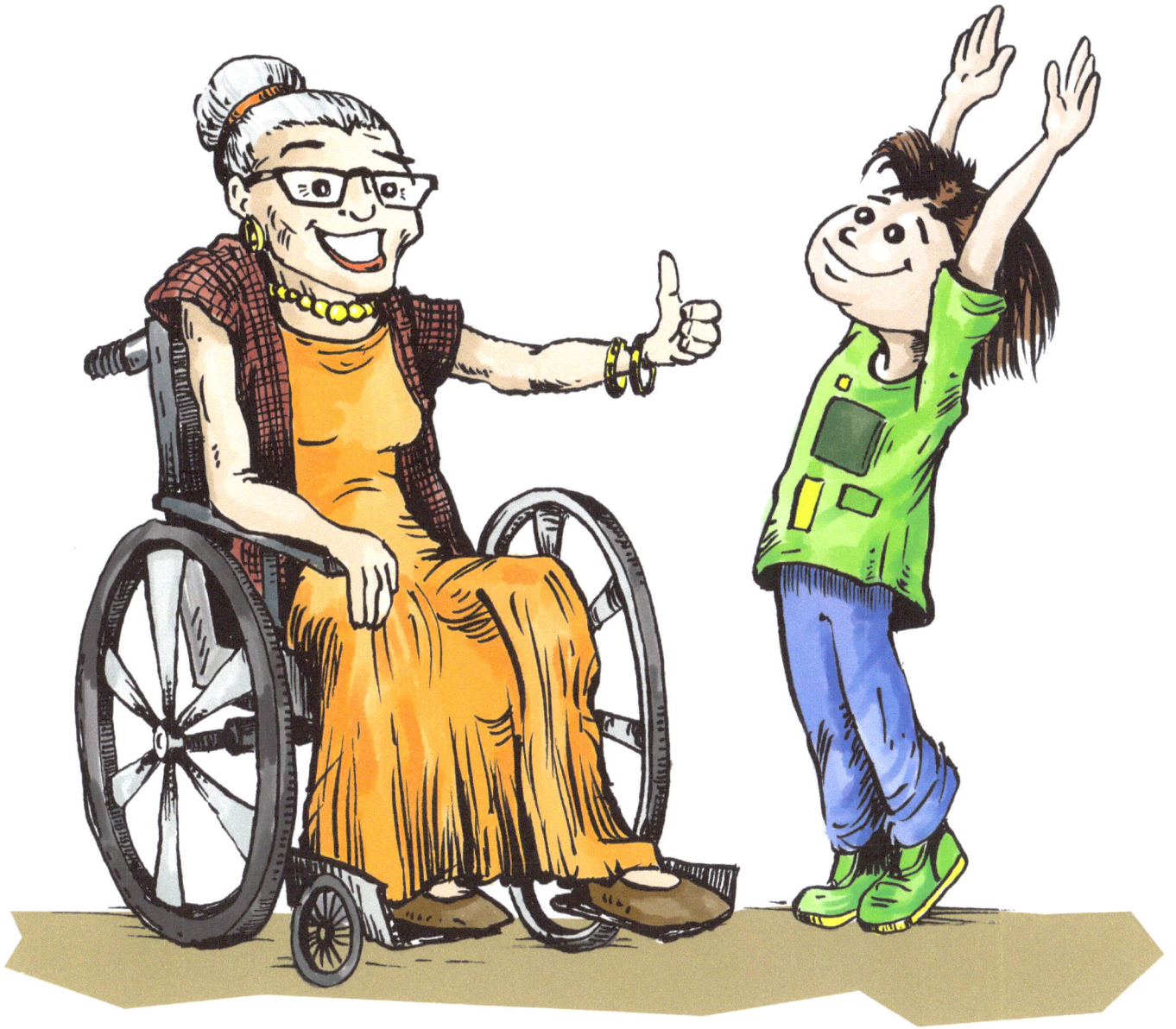

I step back--
Just look at me!

14

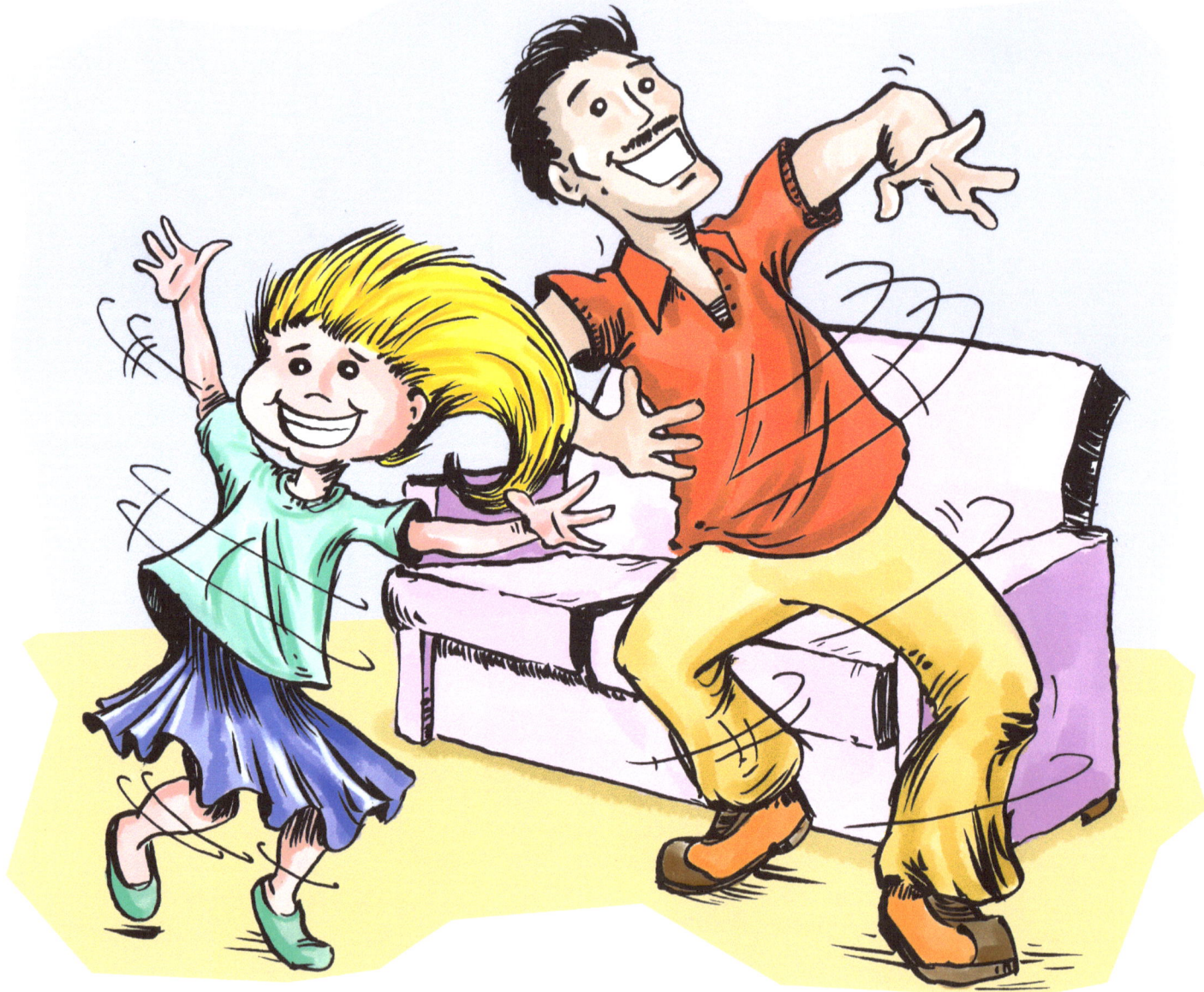

I can move!
Spin! One, Two, Three!

15

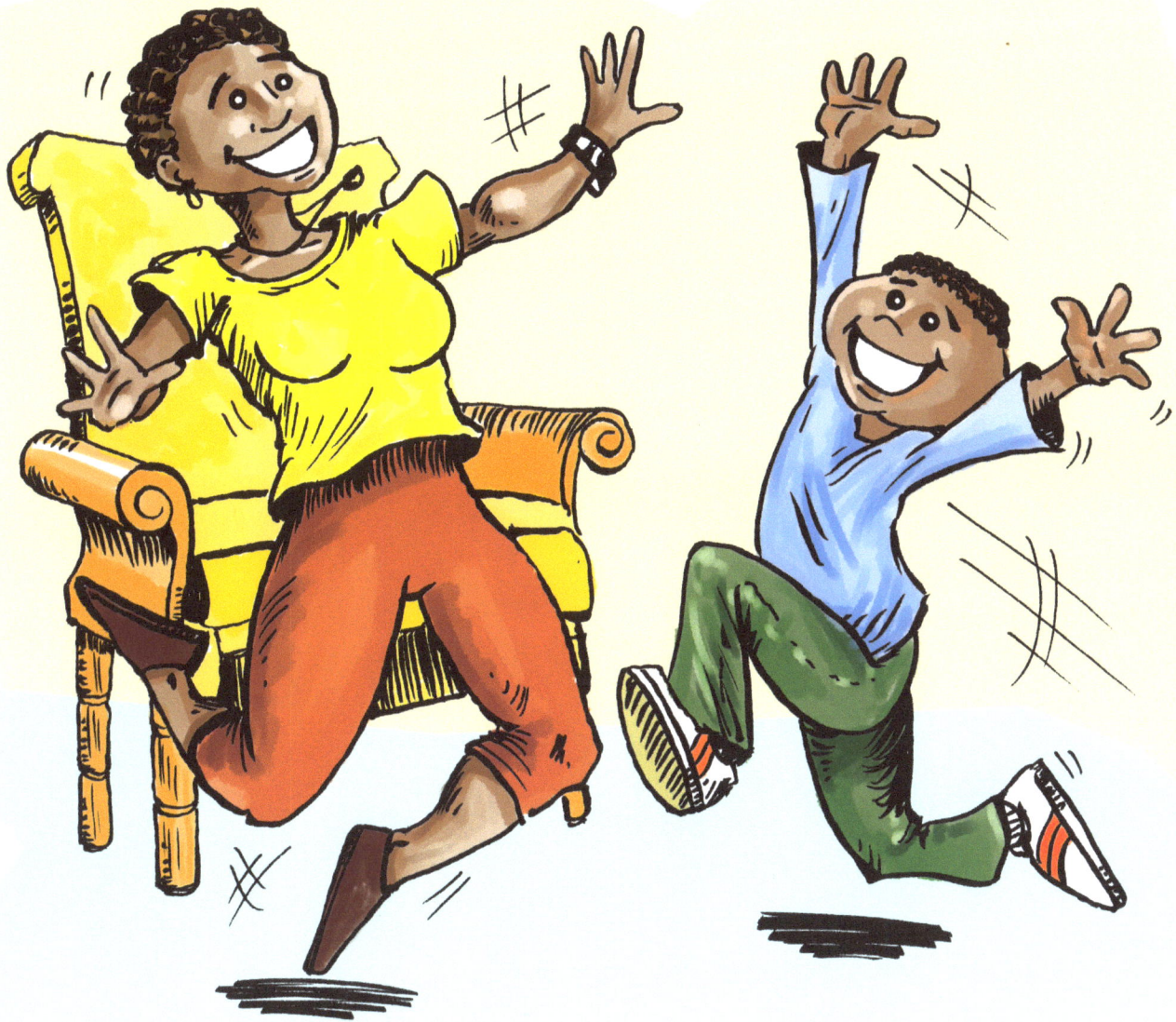

Come on! Get up!
Move with me!

16

I Can Move Activity Chart!

Place a mark or sticker to show you read the page and did the activity.

Day	Jump	Crouch	Run	Walk	March	Lift Knee	Spin
1							
2							
3							
4							
5							
6							
7							
8							
9							
10							
11							
12							
13							
14							

www.ingramcontent.com/pod-product-compliance
Lightning Source LLC
Chambersburg PA
CBHW060856270326
41934CB00002B/159